ADHD
FOR CHILDREN

Learn the best emotional control

strategies to empower your children

Emily Collins

The information provided herein is stated to be truthful and consistent, in that any liability, in terms of inattention or otherwise, by any usage or abuse of any policies, processes, or Instructions contained within is the solitary and utter responsibility of the recipient reader. Under no circumstances will any legal responsibility or blame be held against the publisher for any reparation, damages, or monetary loss due to the information herein, either directly or indirectly. Respective authors own all copyrights not held by the publisher.

The information herein is offered for informational purposes solely and is universal as so. The presentation of the information is without contract or any type of guarantee assurance.

The trademarks that are used are without any consent and the publication of the trademark is without permission or backing by the trademark owner. All trademarks and brands within this book are for clarifying purposes only and are the owned by the owners themselves s, not affiliated with this document.

Table of Contents

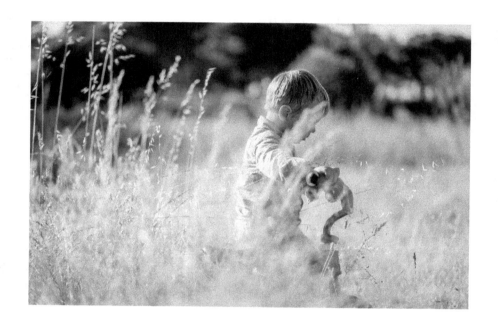

Introduction

ADHD is a neurological disorder characterized by a history of inattention or hyperactive-impulsive behavior that affects normal life in at least two environments, such as school and home. It affects both boys and girls, as well as individuals from all walks of life. The symptoms mentioned above are representative of the wide variety of signs associated with ADHD, but they vary by subtype. ADHD affects about 8.4% of children and 2.5 percent of adults. When a disturbance in the classroom or difficulties with schoolwork occur, ADHD is often found in school-aged children. Adults may be affected as well. It is more prevalent in boys than in females. It's a behavioral wellbeing condition characterized by a slew of chronic issues, including trouble paying attention, hyperactivity, and impulsive behavior. Adult ADHD may cause shaky relationships, weak job or school success, low self-esteem, and a variety of other issues. About the fact that it's called adult ADHD, signs begin in childhood and last until adulthood. ADHD is not often known or identified before an individual is an adult. Adult ADHD signs cannot be as obvious as children's ADHD symptoms.

Hyperactivity in adults can decline, but impulsivity, restlessness, and difficulties paying attention can persist. Adult ADHD therapy is close to childhood ADHD treatment. Medication, psychiatric intervention (psychotherapy), and care with certain co-occurring behavioral wellbeing problems are also part of adult ADHD treatment. The main symptoms of ADHD are inattention and hyperactivity/impulsivity. Some individuals with ADHD struggle with just one of the behaviors, while others struggle with both hyperactivity-impulsivity and inattention. The mixed form of ADHD affects the majority of infants. Hyperactivity is the most prominent ADHD symptom in preschoolers. While some unfocused motor movement, inattention, and impulsivity are common, these activities are more extreme and appear more often in people with ADHD. They obstruct or degrade their ability to act professionally, at college, or at work.

ADHD assessment scales have been used to screen, assess, and monitor the signs of ADHD in both children and adults for almost 50 years. In order to diagnose ADHD in adolescents, rating scales are used. Scales come in a variety of shapes and sizes. ADHD is most often manifested as inattentiveness or hyperactivity-impulsivity. A person with combined form ADHD has six or more symptoms from either type. Almost everybody has any signs related to ADHD at some stage in their life. Whether the problems are new or happened only rarely in the past, you definitely don't have ADHD. Only when diagnoses are serious enough to warrant problems in far more for one area of life is ADHD identified. These bothersome symptoms could be traced all the way back to childhood. Since some ADHD signs are close to those induced by other diseases, such as depression or mood disorders, diagnosing ADHD in adults may be complicated.

DBT guides how to develop self-regulation abilities, which could be useful for people who don't adapt to other methods. Before being adapted to handle adult

ADHD, DBT was used to treat various psychiatric illnesses. It is the brainchild of The Linehan Institute's president, a professor of psychology at the University of Washington. DBT was created to help people with borderline personality disorder cope with social upheavals, like self-harming habits, including cutting (BPD). Unpredictable mood changes and reckless habits, chaotic interactions, acute stress responses, and a persistent likelihood of self-harm and suicide are also symptoms of BPD. If your kid has been diagnosed with ADHD, your doctor has either spoken about or administered ADHD drugs. You may have now discovered that behavioral counseling, also known as behavior change, may be beneficial. Keep in mind that these two treatments are not mutually exclusive choices when you strive to find out the right therapy for your boy. In reality, when it comes to resolving ADHD behavior issues, they always function well together. Medication treatment itself, as well as medication and behavioral therapy together, culminated in the largest change in children's ADHD symptoms, according to the National Institute of

Mental Health. Furthermore, the hybrid therapy was the most effective in reducing ADHD-related oppositional tendencies as well as other aspects of coping, such as relationships with parents and educators.

If you want behavioral treatment instead of medicine because you choose a non-medical solution, your child is too early for medication, or medication has negative side effects, your child will develop emotional, academic, and behavioral skills that can help him manage ADHD over his life. Most children aren't diagnosed with ADHD until they're in kindergarten, but if you think your kid has it until then, it's almost always beneficial (and never harmful) to handle him behaviorally as if he has it. Most people nowadays understand that their minds and bodies are connected in some way. The area of somatic psychotherapy is concerned with the feedback process that exists between the mind and the body, as well as the aspects in which one continually reminds the other. Physical experiences are as essential to somatic therapists as perceptions and emotions are to talk therapists.

Initially, the holistic fusion of body consciousness with classical psychotherapy was utilized to address PTSD by dwelling on the feelings of the body rather than reliving a stressful experience. This method has now been broadened to assist a broader variety of individuals, particularly those with ADHD, in releasing anxiety, apprehension, and rage that may impair their working.

Chapter 1: Getting Started with ADHD Basics

ADHD is a neurological disorder characterized by a history of inattention or hyperactive-impulsive behavior that affects normal life in at least two environments, such as school and home. It affects both boys and girls, as well as individuals from all walks of life. The symptoms mentioned above are representative of the wide variety of signs associated with ADHD, but they vary by subtype. ADHD affects about 8.4% of children and 2.5 percent of adults. When a disturbance in the classroom or difficulties with schoolwork occur, ADHD is often found in school-aged children. Adults may be affected as well. It is more prevalent in boys than in females. It's a behavioral wellbeing condition characterized by a slew of chronic issues, including trouble paying attention, hyperactivity, and impulsive behavior. Adult ADHD may cause shaky relationships, weak job or school success, low self-esteem, and a variety of other issues. About the fact that it's called adult

ADHD, signs begin in childhood and last until adulthood.

ADHD is not often known or identified before an individual is an adult. Adult ADHD signs cannot be as obvious as children's ADHD symptoms. Hyperactivity in adults can decline, but impulsivity, restlessness, and difficulties paying attention can persist. Adult ADHD therapy is close to childhood ADHD treatment. Medication, psychiatric intervention (psychotherapy), and care with certain co-occurring behavioral wellbeing problems are also part of adult ADHD treatment. The main symptoms of ADHD are inattention and hyperactivity/impulsivity. Some individuals with ADHD struggle with just one of the behaviors, while others struggle with both hyperactivity-impulsivity and inattention. The mixed form of ADHD affects the majority of infants.

1.1 ADHD vs. ADD

ADHD was also known as attention deficit disorder (ADD). In the 1990s, that was legally updated. Some people also refer to this one disorder by all terms. The source of ADHD is unknown to experts. It may be caused by a number of factors, including:

- o Genetics. ADHD is a condition that runs in households.

- o Toxic substances. People with ADHD can have an imbalance in brain chemicals.

- o Changes in the brain. Attention-controlling areas of the brain are less involved in children with ADHD.

- o During breastfeeding, poor diet, infections, smoking, alcohol, and drug misuse are all risks. These factors may have an effect on a baby's brain growth.

- o Toxins, such as lead, are a concern. They can have an effect on a child's cognitive growth.

- o A traumatic brain accident or a mental illness. Damage to the frontal lobe of the brain, often known as the prefrontal cortex, may result in difficulties regulating urges and emotions.

ADHD is not caused by sugar. ADHD isn't induced by watching too much TV, having a difficult family life, attending bad classes, or having food allergies.

To parents with ADHD

You may be concerned about transferring the disorder's genes to your kids. Unfortunately, you have no say in whether or not your kid can inherit the ADHD genes. You may, however, choose how attentive you are to your child's possible signs. Be sure your child's pediatrician is aware of your own diagnosis of ADHD. The more you and your child's doctor are informed of early symptoms of ADHD in your child, the better. You should start medication and counseling with your child as soon as possible, which can help him or she learn to deal properly with the effects of ADHD.

1.2 ADHD Rating Scales

ADHD assessment scales have been used to screen, assess, and monitor the signs of ADHD in both children and adults for almost 50 years. In order to diagnose ADHD in adolescents, rating scales are used. Scales come in a variety of shapes and sizes. You or one of the following persons can fill out the forms in the best-case scenario:

- Your kid

- Your parents

- All who look after them

- Educators

- Medical professionals

Scales can help:

- The specialist will do an assessment or diagnosis

- You will be able to track your or your child's growth

- You will be able to consider the larger picture in terms of actions

Scales don't give:

- A full ADHD evaluation

- An impartial view of actions

- Enough proof when used alone

A standard assessment system would include 18 to 90 questions on how many ADHD-related behaviors occur. The questions are focused on the Diagnostic and Statistical Manual of Mental Disorders' concept of ADHD (DSM-5). There are few explanations of these behaviors:

- Having trouble concentrating, planning, and paying attention

- Finding it impossible to sit still

- Trembling

- Twitching

- Finding it impossible to remain careful

- Not being able to wait for one's turn

- Interfering with others

- Experiencing trouble following orders or completing assignments

Since stable children's habits, including squirming and inattention, are normal, scales often inquire for behaviors over the previous six months. It's better to make several people fill out scales because they're arbitrary. It's important to remember that these ADHD assessment scales aren't a formal diagnosis. They do, though, assist doctors in providing one.

What's in a typical ADHD rating scale?

Kids, adolescents, and adults will all use ADHD assessment scales. The time it takes to complete a questionnaire will range from 5 to 20 minutes. You can have them for free or sell them for up to $140 on the internet. While anybody can fill out a rating chart, only the doctor can diagnose ADHD correctly.

- The Infant Behavior Checklist (CBCL), which is for children aged 6 to 18, is a popular ADHD assessment system for children.

- The Vanderbilt Assessment Scale, developed by the National Institute for Children's Health Quality (NICHQ), is for children aged 6 to 12.

- Conners Comprehensive Behavior Rating Scale for children aged 6 to 18 years.

- The Conners-Wells Adolescent Self-Report Scale (for teenagers)

- SNAP-IV (Swanson, Nolan, and Pelham-IV Questionnaire) for children aged 6 to 18.

Some types may divide questions by gender. Boys and girls with ADHD have various traits, such as being hyper and shy, respectively.

Adults may use the following forms:

- Adult ADHD Self-Report Scale (ASRS v1.1)

- BADDS for Adults

- ACDS v1.2 Adult ADHD Clinical Diagnostic Scale

- IV ADHD Rating Scale (ADHD-RS-IV)

Typical questions and scoring system

To assess hyperactivity, a query can probe the level of repetitive talking or fidgeting. Interrupting can be mentioned in impulsivity questions. Hyperactivity, impulsiveness, and inattentiveness may also be measured by rating certain habits. Some assessment measures, such as the SNAP-IV, will often inquire into student success in the classroom. The assessments are structured to search for clear signs of ADHD habits in general.

Rating how much the person:

- ignores tasks or has difficulty finishing up specifics of a project

- interrupts

- is overwhelmed by other items or individuals

- has trouble recalling appointments or duties would be one of the survey questions.

It will rate how many children behave on the go with children. Adults would be able to rate how tough it is for them to relax or unwind. Checklists, reminders, and concerns regarding health history can be used in the adult rating scale. Rating scales will ask you to rate actions on a scale of 0 to 3, or 4 points. Typically, a score of 0 indicates that the condition will never occur, whereas a score of 3 or 4 indicates that it will occur often, and the greater the score, the more serious the symptom. To assess the probability of ADHD, each examination adds up the scores in a particular way. Some claim you require six counted habits to be diagnosed with ADHD, and others say you need to sum up the numbers. Continue reading to learn how certain traditional assessments arrive at their conclusions.

Checklists for adults and children

The CBCL is a program for girls. This questionnaire looks at mental, behavioral, and social issues. It encompasses a wide range of ailments, from autism to anxiety. A shortened guide for signs or effects of ADHD is available from the Centers for Disease Control and Prevention. ADHD is diagnosed when a person exhibits six or more signs of inattention, hyperactivity, or impulsivity. Such signs must be deemed age-inappropriate and have been present for at least six months. Bring the list to a specialist whether your child has a ranking of 6 or more. Be sure another adult, instructor, or caregiver completes the checklist as well. The ASRS v1.1 symptoms guide has

18 queries for adults. Frequency is used to determine the score. When filling out the question, the instructions state that you can think about your job, family, and other social situations.

Scoring the Vanderbilt ADHD Diagnostic Rating Scale

The NICHQ VADS is used by many healthcare practitioners to evaluate ADHD. The scale is intended for children aged 6 to 12, although it may be used by people of any age group if necessary. Parents and teachers can choose from a variety of types. All types test for ADHD and inattention signs. Conduct illness, or antisocial behavior, has its own segment on the parent evaluation scale, whereas intellectual disorders have their own section on the instructor assessment scale. To follow DSM-5's requirements for ADHD, there must be six counted activities with a ranking of 2 or 3 out of 9 questions for inattention or hyperactivity. For the success questions, a score of 4 or higher on two of them, or a score of 5 on one of them, is needed for the results to mean ADHD. Add all of the statistics from the answers and split them by the number of responses if you're using this questionnaire to monitor symptoms. To monitor progress, compare the results of each evaluation.

Scoring the Conners CBRS

The Conners CBRS is used to evaluate children ranging in age from 6 to 18. It's designed to help decide if the pupil needs special education participation or removal, as well as whether the therapy or action is successful.

- Attention deficit hyperactivity disorder (ADHD) is an issue.

- There is a favorable reaction to the care

- Which care options could be the most effective?

There are separate forms for parents, students, and the infant. The short version consists of 25 questions which take between 5 and 1 hour to complete. The extended form is used to assess ADHD and monitor improvement over time. A score of more than 60 indicates ADHD. In contrast, the doctor can translate certain ratings into percentage scores.

Scoring the SNAP-IV Rating Scale

The SNAP-IV has nine questions about inattention and nine questions about hyperactivity and impulsivity. You record the frequency of each item or behavior, ranging from none to a lot. These replies are listed on a scale of 0 to 3. After adding up the points for each section, divide the total by 9 to get the average. Teachers will mark a child who tests higher than 2.56 on the Snap-IV scale as inattentive. The number for parents is 1.78. A ranking of 1.78 for teachers and 1.44 for parents on the hyperactive and impulsive questions shows that ADHD needs to be investigated further.

What happens next?

Diagnosed with ADD [Attention Deficit Disorder] will typically stick around for your child's lifetime, but many reports that ADD [mood swings] issues resolve as he grows older. The disorder is manageable, though.

Standard ADHD therapies include one or more of the following:

- Medication

- Education

- Therapy

- Counseling

Many people (individuals diagnosed with ADHD) undergo medications like Adderall and Ritalin to counter the imbalances in their brain chemistry. Before they prescribe you some cardiac drug, the doctor may have been aware of any issues you may have with the heart as well as any family history with medical complications or that may affect the heart. Check with the doctor to find out any possible adverse effects that could occur. Experts recommend that patients plan a multi-faceted recovery strategy that involves:

- Training and behavioral counseling, as well as coaching

- Refers to the needs of the individual and to their likes and choices

- Is distinguished from other clubs by the fact that it has aims that can be held under surveillance

- Involving families and colleagues in addition to healthcare providers

Any healthcare provider can use rating scales to help determine whether or not anyone has ADHD. Since assessments aren't always constructed to be perfectly unbiased, it is better to enlist people from various sources of varying levels of expertise, like with this example, such as an instructor or a psychiatrist, as opposed to relying on either one to ensure that everyone is well informed. If your tests yield ratings of "ADHD Equal," have an evaluation from a healthcare practitioner, and your scores match, follow the professional's advice.

1.3 Challenges of Identifying ADHD

ADHD is a progressive neurodevelopmental disease that affects 11% of children in kindergarten. In upwards of 75 percent of cases, the disorder's signs last until adulthood. Inappropriate forms of hyperactivity, inattention, and impulsivity are among these signs. During school and kindergarten development, it is the most often diagnosed psychiatric illness. Although signs of ADHD can occur in the development of a "typical" infant, parents should be aware of whether these signs are interfering with everyday life or are severe. The frequency, intensity, and duration of these symptoms, as well as how often they interfere with both the child's ability to cope in life, are what contribute to these symptoms being labeled as "ADHD." We deem it a 'disorder'—in this situation, ADHD—when signs are severe for age and conflict with major life events on a routine basis. It may be difficult to get a correct diagnosis of ADHD. According to another doctor, this may be attributed to a lack of thorough testing to rule out other neurological or wellbeing problems that could be mistaken for ADHD. Since inattention or hyperactivity is a sign or result of almost all other behavioral health conditions, the difficulty is ensuring that your physician has considered options such that such diagnoses are not confused for ADHD. ADHD in children and adolescents is currently challenging to detect.

Making an ADHD diagnosis in preschoolers is perhaps the most complex. Many of the habits that make up the disorder's main manifestations, or diagnosis characteristics, overlap with the usual spectrum of behavior.

According to researchers, it is important for people to realize that ADHD can be present on any continent.

This has prompted researchers to conclude that the disease is not exacerbated by poor living conditions, social media, or tv viewing.

It is a biomedical disease that often necessitates medical attention.

Although, thankfully, we will assist the vast number of children and adults in being even more functional and reducing their struggles.

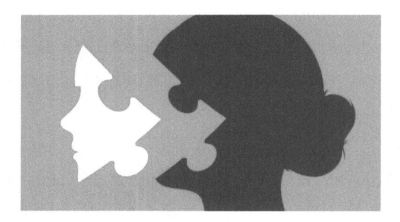

ADHD May Affect Certain Brain Regions in Kids

An expansion of the brain regions involved in action occurs with children with kids who have ADHD, claim the researchers. Recent research that examined brain structure in children with respect to determining whether there was a connection to attention loss or hyperactivity has found has discovered that regions with decreased volume in the former as mentioned in the recent Journal of the International Neuropsychology review, that is, according to researchers, which looked at the mental growth in the range of children between the ages of 4 and 5, significant increases in mental abilities occurred. Experts from the Kennedy Krieger Institute in Baltimore used both behavior and cognitive testing, as well as functional magnetic resonance imaging, to evaluate the children with ADHD. Among these children, 52 who did not take medicine, they measured their brain growth with both high-resolution MRI and cognitive tests and imaging. Children with ADHD showed a reduction in brain volume in various areas or fields, as compared to children who did not have symptoms. They have indicated that people with symptoms have much less grey matter capacity. The areas of the brain that saw the greatest declines in patients of ADHD symptoms were those that are essential for psychological-behavioral regulation, as well as the certainty of behavioral symptoms. The research was the first of its type to concentrate on preschool-aged children and brain volume, despite the fact that several reports have concentrated on ADHD in school-aged children. Finding signs of ADHD with an MRI scan may be beneficial for children in establishing a "biomarker" for the condition. "Studying behavior and brain growth of preschool children with signs of ADHD is important since we often see manifestations of the condition in this age group, if not earlier. The sooner we can recognize 'biomarkers' of the disease, the more we will be able to identify early and more focused treatments that will potentially minimize the disorder's later risks."

1.4 Future of ADHD Research

To better explain the condition, researchers expect to track the kids from the sample across their childhood and early adolescence. Researchers expect that by observing these children from an early age, they would be able to figure out which initial brain and behavioral signs are more closely linked to subsequent challenges, or, perhaps better, which features of early growth may indicate a better result and rehabilitation from the disorder. At various ages, ADHD may have a different effect on one's quality of life. Although many parents are concerned about the academic consequences of ADHD-related behavioral issues, there are an amount of other important aspects to consider that go beyond the school years. ADHD can increase the likelihood of injury in small children, as well as social and peer interactions as they grow older, siblings or family relations, risk-taking habits, and the harmful effects that can result, such as bad driving and crashes, sexual results, or early parenthood, and a greater risk of drug misuse. ADHD in adults may have a negative impact on work results, money planning, marital strife, and divorce possibility. Functional characteristics of ADHD have been studied extensively, but as such, much further research needs to be done on the biological causes; ADHD has many causes and complications that are yet to be discovered. Experts are optimistic that the research would help to reduce the harmful effects of ADHD. We may continue to incorporate tailored, preventative treatments in young children with the intention of mitigating harmful effects or even correcting the trajectory of this disease through understanding the minds of children who develop into the illness as well as those who grow out of it by knowing the brains of children that grow into disorder as well as those who grow out of it.

1.5 Combined Type ADHD

A neurodevelopmental disease is known as attention deficit hyperactivity disorder. It's most often diagnosed in infants, but it may also affect adults. Symptoms are normally classified into one of the following groups:

- inattention, or a lack of desire to concentrate

- hyperactivity-impulsivity, or the failure to sit still or maintain the power of one's behavior

Both signs are seen in the majority of infants. ADHD mixed form is another name for this condition. Continue reading to find out more about mixed form ADHD and how to handle it.

What are the symptoms and signs of combined type ADHD?

ADHD is most often manifested as inattentiveness or hyperactivity-impulsivity. A person with combined form ADHD has six or more symptoms from either type.

Inattentiveness Symptoms

Examples of inattentive behavior can include symptoms like:

- Failing to obey directions

- Pretending to not respond and being quickly distracted

- Missing or recalling items or activities

- Being easily overwhelmed

- Having trouble carrying through with projects or duties

- Daydreaming or failure to pay attention

Hyperactivity and Impulsivity Symptoms

The below are the most prominent symptoms and signs of hyperactivity and impulsivity:

- fidgeting or squirming

- inability to sit still for long stretches of time

- nonstop conversation

- bouncing across the bed

- doing something that isn't right without thought

- being irritable or disrespectful

- interfering with or interrupting other people's interactions

- having trouble waiting for your turn

Six or more of these symptoms, as well as six or more signs of inattentiveness, are present in an individual with combined form ADHD.

How is ODD linked to ADHD?

When the kid or teen displays a history of resistance to you or another authority figure, this is known as opposition defiance disorder (ODD). ODD affects around 40% of children with ADHD. The habits may be linked to the ADHD form of hyperactivity or impulsivity. It may also be a way for children with ADHD to deal with frustration or mental tension. Rage, irritability, outbursts, and defiance are common symptoms of ODD. A kid with ODD can even have an argumentative disposition or partake in obnoxious habits on purpose. Behavioral medication may aid in the treatment of ODD symptoms.

What increases your risk for combined-type ADHD?

Causes

While the mechanisms of ADHD are likely to be the same among both forms, research has yet to discover one. However, some research has discovered a number of possible causes that can affect a person's chance of developing ADHD. Environmental influences, for example, can play a role.

Risk factors

According to another report, multiple genes may increase the risk of developing ADHD.

Inherited genes

ADHD has been shown to run in households, according to one report.

Toxin exposure during infancy or pregnancy

Toxin exposure, such as lead, can increase a child's risk of developing ADHD.

Traumatic brain injury

A limited percentage of children with traumatic brain injuries experience ADHD.

Alcohol or tobacco use during pregnancy

Pregnant women who smoke raise their child's chance of having ADHD, according to a report from Washington University School of Medicine.

During breastfeeding, drinking alcohol and consuming medications may raise a child's chance of developing the condition.

Low-birth weight or premature delivery

According to a report published in the journal Pediatrics, babies delivered past their due date have a higher risk of developing ADHD later in life.

Gender

CDC reports that boys are more than twice as likely to experience ADHD than children.

What to expect at your doctor's?

There is no single examination that will determine whether or not anyone has ADHD. Both forms of ADHD are diagnosed in the same manner by a doctor or clinician. And there are several differences in the requirements for mixed form ADHD. Your psychiatrist can search at six or more signs with all hyperactivity and impulsiveness inattentiveness forms if you have mixed type ADHD.

What your doctor will do?

To rule out other problems, the doctor will first administer a detailed medical review. Any conditions, such as developmental disabilities and anxiety disorders, may be mistaken for ADHD. Then they'll look for signs correlated with ADHD subtypes in your infant. This might include keeping an eye on your child throughout the day. Many other ADHD rating scales can be completed by both you and your kids. These may be used by the specialist to aid with the assessment or diagnosis. These scales do not have a conclusive solution; however, they will assist you and your doctor in gaining a better understanding of the larger picture. The questionnaires will inquire into your child's actions at school, at home, and in other situations. Requesting behavior descriptions from those that work with your infants, such as educators and other family and friends, will help you see a bigger picture about your child's behavior.

How do you treat combined type ADHD?

Medicine

Medications for ADHD may help the child's inattention, cognitive impairment, and hyperactivity. They can also aid in the development of physical control.

Stimulants

Psychostimulants are often used by doctors. These may assist with the behavioral symptoms of ADHD and make it easier to concentrate on daily activities. The medications function by boosting brain chemicals involved in cognition and focus. When used as intended, psychostimulants are healthy for both you and your kids. They could have adverse consequences in some situations.

If you or your child has a pre-existing health disorder or is experiencing stimulant side effects such as:

- loss of appetite

- sleeping disorders, consult your doctor.

- the tics

- alterations in appearance

- irritability or fear

- Abdominal ache

- throbbing pains

Non-stimulant drugs

If stimulants don't operate, the doctor will recommend something else. These drugs take longer to function, but they can help with ADHD symptoms. Antidepressants may also help with ADHD symptoms. Antidepressants, though, are yet to be accepted as a medication by the Food and Drug Administration.

Psychotherapy

Children, particularly those aged 6 to 12, benefit from a combination of therapy and medication. Research further suggests that therapeutic methods and treatments for children and youth with ADHD are highly effective.

Behavioral therapy

The purpose of this therapy is to assist with behavior modification. It instills in you and your child the importance of positive behaviors. An adult, instructor, or educator should use behavioral counseling to help a child develop healthy habits. Parent preparation, classroom supervision, peer reinforcement, organizational training, or a mixture of these therapies can be used in behavior modification.

Cognitive-behavioral therapy (CBT)

CBT helps people with communication skills to help them change unwanted

behaviors and manage their anxiety and depression symptoms. While there is limited research on CBT and ADHD, early evidence suggests that it could be helpful for adults with the disorder. However, these therapies must be more precise and refined.

Family therapy

Relations with parents and relatives may be impacted by ADHD, particularly before anyone is diagnosed. Family counseling will help everyone learn to deal with and treat the effects of ADHD in a family member. It can also assist in family cohesion and connectivity.

What techniques can help someone with combined ADHD?

For children

The importance of structural support for children with ADHD cannot be overstated. A child's symptoms should be managed with organization and continuity. Together, you and your child can:

- assist with the development of a routine and timetable

- prepare for schedule shifts as far in advance as practicable.

- Create a method of management such that everything has a location.

- Follow the laws exactly.

- praising and rewarding positive leadership

If your kid has ADHD, you should still promote positive behavior by:

- restricting options when your child has to choose

- minimizing disruptions when they are performing a task

- assisting them with developing a healthier lifestyle

- Providing fun opportunities for your child by things he or she loves and excels at.

For adults

Adults may develop teamwork and life management skills when working with a therapist or psychologist that will help in:

- establishing and sustaining a schedule

- being used to making and utilizing lists

- making use of reminders

- cutting down big programs or activities into smaller chunks

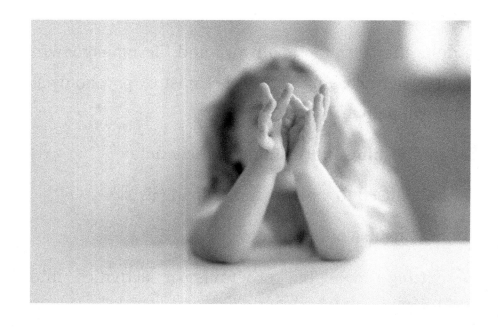

Chapter 2: Developing Knowledge and Busting Myths

A student experiencing inattentive ADHD might silently gaze out the window as her work piles up; this spacey or daydreamy behavior is sometimes ignored or misinterpreted as laziness or apathy. Symptoms of inattentive ADHD are much less likely to be identified by caregivers, students, and care practitioners, according to the National Institute of Mental Health, and they are poorly treated.

This will contribute to a lifetime of intellectual discontent, apathy, and guilt. The DSM-V, the diagnostic manual for ADHD published by the American Psychiatric Association, describes nine signs of inattentive ADHD. To warrant a diagnosis in a child or teenager, at least six of these must be apparent and seriously disrupt the patient's life. Students with inattentive ADHD are only relayed about half of the commands orally, if at all. They have more doodles than documents in their journals, and they will need to document and listen to lectures many times to fully comprehend the material. Cocktail parties are not just for adults. They disrupt other people's tales with their own stories, forget people's names, and fall asleep in the middle of any discussion. ADHD is a neurological disorder characterized by a history of inattention or hyperactive-impulsive behavior that affects normal life in at least two environments, such as school and home. It affects both boys and girls, as well as individuals from all walks of life. The symptoms mentioned above are representative of the wide variety of signs associated with ADHD, but they vary by subtype.

From time to time, everybody loses their keys or phone. People experiencing inattentive ADHD also tell each other about having their spectacles in the fridge or peas in their pocket.

They have a habit of misplacing the necessities of life on a regular basis, such as keys, wallets, backpacks, and sports accessories. It could be a warning if you've discovered that you need a "launch pad" by the door to guarantee you don't lose your phone and can't live without any of the locator systems attached to your keychain.

2.1 Time Management, Emotional Regulation, Anxiety, and Focus

Consider hundreds of vehicles entering a crosswalk with no traffic lights or stop signs. Each day, the prefrontal cortex of the ADHD brain is unable to adequately control the different thoughts and emotions when various vehicles pass the intersection. Discover more about the ADHD "Intersection Model." Most ADHD patients are full of misinformation concerning concentration deficiency disorder (ADHD or ADD). Many people believe that taking drugs alone can help them manage their symptoms. Others feel that after they have finished college, ADHD would have little effect on their lives. And absolutely no one really comprehends how the ADHD brain acts to trigger the effects they do. To that end, experts have created the Intersection Model, a paradigm that can be applied in a person's life to help them make sense of their actions, desires, and feelings, as well as build techniques to control them.

ADHD and the Prefrontal Cortex

The prefrontal cortex is at the heart of the intersection model (PFC). It is in charge of dreaming, analyzing thoughts, and controlling behavior. This involves resolving contradictory emotions, making moral decisions, and anticipating the likely consequences of acts or incidents. This crucial part of the brain controls both short- and long-term decision-making. Furthermore, the PFC aids in mind control, allowing individuals to pay attention, read, and reflect on their objectives. In this design, the PFC serves as a crossroads for focus, actions, judgment, and emotional reactions, which experts refer to as "cars" or "messages." An individual experiencing ADHD is likely to respond to whatever is currently occupying his attention, such as a quicker car or a more powerful tweet. The PFC is unchecked in people with ADHD; there are no traffic signals or stop signs from monitoring which message (car) gets through first. You may be the brightest, most inspired student in the world, yet if the instructor says, "This type of dog..." and your first reaction is, "I guess what my pet is doing right now?" you would get overwhelmed.

ADHD and Focus

This uncontrolled convergence could be the reason for your concentration wandering. Assume you're washing up in the kitchen and come across everything that belongs upstairs. When you head down the stairwell, you get annoyed by the piled laundry in the living room. You might say to yourself, "I forgot to do that," and go straight to folding laundry, oblivious to the fact that you were supposed to be going up the stairs, not to mentioned washing up the kitchen. Individuals with ADHD get overwhelmed when something is now occupying their attention blocks out other, less important signals. This can arise in the middle of a discussion where a word prompts a thought that moves to a completely different subject.

ADHD and Time Management

The PFC is also where judgment is made. It's a judgment decision when you think, "That'll take me 5 minutes to complete." It's still a judgment call to say, "I'll be there in a half hour." We can't see or sense time. The emotion associated with a monitoring stage or an unresolved job sends a stronger message to the ADHD brain than understanding or conceptualizing time. "Don't speak to me, I have so many things to do and no time to do them!" an individual with ADHD might exclaim when faced with a deadline. Or the individual tells himself, "This job will take forever," and then uses it as an excuse to put off doing it. The job will take about 10 minutes if the individual just got underway. In this scenario, the feeling behind the estimate of how long it would take to reach the deadline is the fastest vehicle in the intersection.

ADHD and Emotional Regulation

Emotion's flow into the PFC junction, causing rapid mood shifts. "Ten minutes ago, I won the lottery." Isn't it fantastic? However, my sink is already overflowing. Why does this happen to me every time?" Impulsive rage (or sorrow, or happiness, or worry) seems to appear out of nowhere, but it is simply a quick response to a recent incident (in this case, the sink debacle). And that's what is occupying the person's attention at the time. The quicker car in the ADHD brain is whatever feeling is in view at the time. This explains why people with ADHD have a tendency to show feelings more strongly than is appropriate in a particular environment. This emotional expression is often undiagnosed as a mood disturbance in females with ADHD.

ADHD and Behavior/Impulsivity

Individuals with ADHD self-medicate or overspend on frivolous goods in search of immediate satisfaction rather than larger, longer-lasting benefits. They can cling to a technique even after it has been proven ineffective, rushing through tasks and making mistakes as a result of their hurry. Bad criticism from the outside environment, behavioral challenges, and work or academic problems all result from this mindset. Such rigidity and hyperactivity have a demoralizing and isolating impact over time. As a result, the person having ADHD develops a mentality that emphasizes the drawbacks, exacerbating the issue. When we suggest things like, "Nothing is going to get better, so why try to be friends?" or "They're not supposed to like me anymore, so why try to be friends?" It can trigger us to give up trying when we believe the case can only result in disappointment.

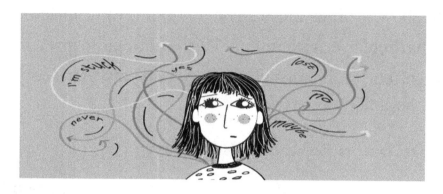

Being consistently late is aided by the quicker automobile metaphor. You would be late to work if you think to yourself on the way out the door, "I have 15 minutes remaining, I will only do this one thing." You would pause to say, "Wow, I have 15 minutes, but that's not enough time to do this stuff, or I'll be late to work like last time," if you didn't have ADHD. If you have ADHD, the better meaning isn't that you were late for work the last time, but more that you want to play a video game for a few minutes or call a buddy to head out on the weekend right now. And you're running late for work once again. Since your precious memories are being cut short from what is now occupying your attention, you keep repeating the same stuff over and over.

ADHD and Anxiety

The overwhelming number of people experiencing an ADHD nervous system is not overly impulsive. They are hyperactive. The majority of individuals with untreated ADHD have four to five problems going on in their heads at the same time. People experiencing untested/untreated ADHD are believed to compensate for their challenges through experiencing anxiety-like symptoms such as rushing impulses, sleep problems, nervousness, and constant concern. This overcompensation may take the form of When you drive to work, you wonder aloud, "Did the garage door really close?" I don't recall having it up close before. What if I pushed something and the garage door opened because the sensor was tripped? A robber may note that there are no vehicles in the garage and nobody at home. He's coming in and steal everything I own. He'll even allow the cats out before he goes. I don't think I'll ever see them again. I adore them and couldn't imagine my life without them. I'll have to double-check. However, I would be late for work. "How am I having to discuss this to my boss?" As we previously said, individuals with ADHD are prone to forgetting objects that aren't in their immediate concentration, so these nervous feelings are an effort to hold certain objects (cars) in the junction, so the individual doesn't worry about them. Doing a lot on your mind causes a lot of anxiety, like a traffic jam. You're likely to get anxiously frustrated and shut down if so many objects — feelings or impulses — want and push across the junction at the same moment. For example, you don't understand what to do first while cleaning a cluttered space with several things vying for your attention, with none of them standing out as more relevant than the others because you don't understand what to do first. When you head to the supermarket for paper towels and return back with all except paper towels, it's aggravating. When you walk into the shop, purchasing paper towels is the quickest car, yet if you see the delicious-looking spaghetti salad or the gleaming red apples, they overshadow the towels; unless you've put "buy paper towels" on a shopping list and read it.

2.2 ADHD Symptoms in Girls and Women

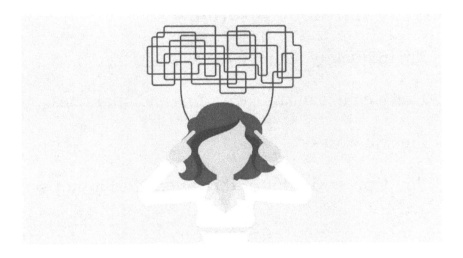

The signs of ADHD in women and girls may be very distinct. As a result, counselors have developed a guide for girls with ADHD symptoms. Since girls feel ADHD more emotionally than boys, who get recognition for unruly behavior, it can be figured out by girls themselves, not guardians or instructors. Most of the counselors' concerns are relevant to boys because they deal with productivity issues, general inattention, hyperactivity, impulsivity, and sleeping issues. The following comments, on the other hand, are aimed specifically at females, and each one must be replied with Clearly Agreed, Agreed, Doubtful, Disagreed, and Disagree Strongly:

Anxiety and Mood Disorders

- I'm frequently tempted to weep.

- I get a couple of stomach pains and migraines.

- I'm still worried.

- I'm depressed a lot of the time, and I'm not sure why.

School Anxiety

- I hate getting named on by the instructor because I sometimes don't pay attention in class.

- If I don't understand what the instructor wants us to do in class, I feel humiliated.

- I don't lift my hand or volunteer in class except though I have anything to suggest.

Social-Skill Deficits

- Other girls don't really like me, and I'm not sure exactly.

- I have disagreements with my friends.

- I don't know how to handle or speak to a group of girls when I try to join them.

- I sometimes feel left out.

Emotional Over-Reactivity

- I'm more likely than other girls to get my feelings hurt.

- My emotions fluctuate a lot.

- I'm more irritable and enraged than most girls.

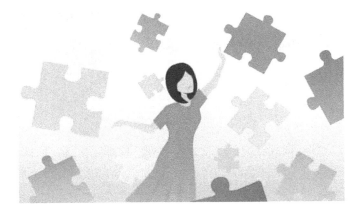

And if an infant meets all of the medical requirements for ADHD, he or she does not have the condition. A clinician must see convincing proof that the effects decrease the quality of social, educational, or job-related functioning before making a conclusive diagnosis. If a girl fits the medical requirements but may not have ADHD, her parents may look at other possibilities. Maybe she's only a little "motivated." Maybe she isn't eating well or doing sufficiently. Alternatively, the boy may be suffering from one or even more "look-alike" disorders such as autism, oppositional defiant disorder, and intellectual disabilities. Food allergies, hearing problems, or an environmental reaction, as well as other psychiatric problems like auditory processing impairment, sensory integration disorder, and perhaps a mood disorder, may cause signs similar to ADHD symptoms.

Chapter 3: ADHD Natural Treatments and Interventions

Several psychosocial therapies have been found to aid victims and their friends in coping with symptoms and improving daily functioning. In addition, in order to achieve their maximum capacity and excel, children and adults experiencing ADHD need support and guidance from their parents, friends, and teachers. Frustration, blame, and rage could have developed up inside a home before a child has been diagnosed, particularly in school-aged children. To resolve negative emotions, parents and children can need professional assistance. Parents will learn regarding ADHD and how it impacts their families from mental health providers. They can often assist the infant and his or her family in learning different abilities, habits, and means of communicating with one another. ADHD can be managed in a variety of ways. But even so, research suggests that for certain children, a multimodal approach is the best approach to manage symptoms. This implies a well-coordinated collection of treatment methods.

All of the symptoms of ADHD may be alleviated with medication and recovery. Psychologists, physicians, parents and students, must all work closely. ADHD drugs help many patients suppress hyperactivity and impulsivity while still improving their capacity to concentrate, function, and understand. Medication may also help in muscle coordination. A few different prescriptions or dosages may need to be tested before an individual finds the one that fits well for them. The prescribing doctor must keep a close eye on everyone who is taking drugs. In recent decades, the development of drugs to manage ADHD has skyrocketed. According to the Ce for CDC, the number of children diagnosed with ADHD rose by 41% between 2003 and 2011. As of 2011, it was reported that 11% of kids between the ages of 4 and 17 had been diagnosed with ADHD. That's a total of 6.4 million kids. There are some more normal choices if you don't want to cure this condition with medications.

By stimulating and regulating neurotransmitters, ADHD medications may help to alleviate symptoms. Neurotransmitters are molecules that send messages from your brain to your body's nerves. Clinical studies are research experiments that examine alternative methods for preventing, diagnosing, and treating illnesses and disorders. Clinical studies are used to see whether an experimental test or medication is effective and secure. While individuals may profit from participating in a research trial, subjects should be mindful that the primary goal of a clinical study is to learn new research expertise such that prospective patients may be better served. Many trials with patients and safe participants are studied by researchers at NIMH and across the world. For what clinical trials revealed years before, we already have fresh and improved care choices. Be a part of the medical breakthroughs of the future. Consult the doctor about research experiments, their advantages and disadvantages, and whether they are suitable for you. ADHD, or attention deficit hyperactivity disorder, is a developmental disorder that may last into adulthood.

In 2011, about 11% of children aged 4 to 17 in the United States were diagnosed with ADHD. ADHD symptoms may be disruptive in some situations or also in a child's daily life. They can struggle to regulate their attitudes and feelings at college or in social situations. This could have an effect on their growth or academic performance. In its heart, it is a self-control disease, and controlling impulses is only one aspect of it. Children with ADHD usually have an inherent inhibition problem that has a detrimental effect on executive performance. Our brain's self-management mechanism, executive functioning assists us in planning, completing tasks, and regulating our emotions.

3.1 Supplements and Herbs for ADHD

Supplements

Supplements can help to alleviate the symptoms of ADHD. These supplements contain the following:

- Vitamin B-6

- Zinc

- Magnesium

- L-carnitine

The findings, however, have been mixed. Passionflower, ginseng, and Ginkgo are some of the herbs that can assist with hyperactivity. Supplementing without a doctor's supervision is risky, particularly in infants. If you're interested in exploring some natural treatments, talk to the doctor. They will order a blood test to determine your child's existing amounts of a nutrient before they begin taking supplements.

Herbs and Supplements for ADHD

ADHD, or attention deficit hyperactivity disorder, is a developmental disorder that may last into adulthood. In 2011, about 11% of children aged 4 to 17 in the United States were diagnosed with ADHD. ADHD symptoms may be disruptive in some situations or also in a child's daily life. They can struggle to regulate their attitudes and feelings at college or in social situations. This could have an effect on their growth or academic performance. The following are examples of ADHD behaviors:

- Becoming easily distracted

- Feeling impatient often

- Not following directions

- Fidgety

To relieve ADHD effects, the child's doctor will administer drugs such as stimulants or antidepressants. They can even refer your child to a counselor who specializes in this region. Alternative therapies for ADHD effects might be of concern to you as well. Before attempting a new alternative therapy, consult a doctor. They will explain the advantages and disadvantages of using that in your child's care schedule.

Supplements for ADHD

According to certain findings, some dietary products may help with ADHD symptoms.

Zinc

Zinc is a trace mineral that is important for brain wellbeing. A zinc deficiency can have an effect on the brain's ability to work properly. Zinc supplements, according to the Mayo Clinic, can help with hyperactivity, impulsivity, and social issues. However, further research is needed. Zinc supplementation can only be useful in people who have a significant risk of zinc deficiency, according to a study of zinc and ADHD. Zinc-rich foods are as follows:

- oysters

- poultry

- dairy products

- red meat

- fortified cereals

- beans

- whole grains

Omega-3 fatty acids

If your child doesn't have enough omega-3 from his or her diet, a supplement can be beneficial. The research results on the advantages are mixed. Omega-3 fatty acids may influence the movement of serotonin and dopamine in the frontal cortex of the brain. DHA is an omega-3 fatty acid that is essential for brain development. DHA levels in people with ADHD are usually smaller than in people without the disorder. DHA and other omega-3 fatty acids can be used in fatty fish, such as:

- salmon

- halibut

- anchovies

- tuna

- herring

- mackerel

Omega-3 fatty acid supplements, according to the NCCIH, can help with ADHD symptoms. According to the Mayo Clinic, certain children can take 200 milligrams of omega-3 flaxseed oil and 25 milligrams of vitamin C supplementation twice a day for three months. However, the evidence for flaxseed oil's efficacy in treating ADHD is mixed.

Iron

According to some studies, there is a correlation between ADHD and low iron levels. According to a 2012 report, iron deficiency in children and young adults can increase the risk of mental health disorders. Iron is needed for the development of dopamine and norepinephrine. These neurotransmitters aid in the regulation of the reward system, impulses, and tension in the brain. Supplements can be beneficial if your child's iron levels are poor. According to the National Center for Complementary and Integrative Health, iron supplementation may help people with ADHD who are iron deficient. However, so much iron may be harmful. Before adding iron supplements to your child's diet, consult with their specialist.

Magnesium

Another essential mineral for brain wellbeing is magnesium. Moodiness, sensory confusion, and a reduced attention span are all symptoms of magnesium deficiency. Magnesium supplementation, on the other hand, could be ineffective if your kid does not have a magnesium deficit. There are still several reports about how magnesium supplementation impacts ADHD symptoms. Before including magnesium supplements in any care plan for your boy, consult with his or her doctor. Magnesium may be harmful in large concentrations, causing nausea, diarrhea, and cramps. You should get enough magnesium by eating a healthy diet. Magnesium-rich diets contain the following:

- dairy products

- beans

- whole grains

- leafy greens

Melatonin

Sleep issues are a known side effect of ADHD. While melatonin does not help with ADHD symptoms, it does help with sleep regulation, particularly in those who suffer from chronic insomnia. Melatonin was shown to increase sleep time in 105 add children between the ages of 6 and 12. Over the course of four weeks, these children were given 3 to 6 milligrams of melatonin 30 minutes before bedtime.

Herbs for ADHD

Herbal therapies are often used for treating ADHD. Just since they are herbal does not suggest they are always more successful than conventional medications. Here are some of the herbs commonly used in ADHD therapy.

Korea ginseng

Observational research sought to determine the efficacy of Korean red ginseng use in the treatment of children with ADHD. At the end of eight weeks, these experiments, it seems that red ginseng will help mitigate hyperactivity. However, additional study is required.

Valerian root and lemon balm

An analysis of 169 children with ADHD examined the valerian root and lemon balm extracts separately to try to understand their distinct effects on the child's conduct. In seven weeks, their attention decreased from 75% to 14%, their hyperactivity (or: impulsive behavior) decreased from 61%, and after that, they completed the program, the impulse to behave had fallen from 59% to 16% Self-person attributes such as socialization, sleeping, and the stress of symptoms have increased. You will be able to purchase valerian root and lemon balm extracts online.

Ginkgo biloba

There's no evidence to support that the claims that Ginkgo Biloba is useful for ADHD, nor is there evidence to disprove them. To some extent, it lacks the effectiveness of conventional therapies, but it is unknown whether it works better than placebo. According to the NCCI, there is not enough data to support this herb for attention-deficit disorder. Taking extra Ginkgo Biloba (Gingko extract is a) raises the chance of bleeding, so seek medical advice before use.

St. John's wort

While several people use this herb to treat ADHD, there is no proof that it is more effective than a placebo.

Talk to your doctor

Before seeking some new supplements or natural medicine, consult your doctor. What works with other people may or may not work for you. Any dietary herbal remedies and supplements can interfere with other medicines you or your child are taking. Dietary improvements, in addition to vitamins and herbs, can help with ADHD symptoms. Remove items that cause hyperactivity from your child's diet. Foods containing artificial colors and ingredients, such as sodas, fruit juices, and vividly colored cereals, fall under this category.

3.2 Assist Children with ADHD in Managing Emotional Outpourings

Identify why children with ADHD are challenged.

In its heart, it is a self-control disease, and controlling impulses is only one aspect of it. Children with ADHD usually have an inherent inhibition problem that has a detrimental effect on executive performance. Our brain's self-management mechanism, executive functioning assists us in planning, completing tasks, and regulating our emotions.

Take into account their developmental stage.

Children with ADHD may have executive performance that varies between their development level and those of kids two-thirds their age. As a result, where their children are having difficulty controlling their feelings at the moment, parents should act based on their developmental stage rather than their age. A kid who is ten years old and acts like a six-year-old, for example, should be treated as a six-year-old.

Value consistency and stability

Limits, schedules, and household guidelines should all be compatible. Posting these around the home can also be beneficial. Furthermore, if your child is irritated when prompted to do anything that isn't in the schedule, either-or statements may improve.

Provide assistance where they are most likely to need it

Determine whether your child is more likely to have a breakdown. Experts recommend setting in motion strategies to improve external executive processing deficiency at the time and place when he is having the most difficulty.

Assist them in comprehending their emotions

It is critical to assist children in comprehending their thoughts such that they can continue to recognize and articulate their inner feelings. This will help them respond with phrases instead of raw anger and physical violence in the long run.

Many youngsters, for example, struggle to get up for the day, and repeated prompts often result in an epic meltdown. Rather than providing written instructions, have a list of pictures in her room of what she wants to do for the day, such as get ready, clean her teeth, and put on shoes.

Respond peacefully in the spur of the moment.

It's impossible to be cool in the face of uncertainty. Rising our voices, voicing aggressive sentiment, and speaking with a rough tone, on the other hand, is like pouring kerosene on a fire that is already burning. We consider doing something along the lines of, "I see you're mad." We should talk about it until you've calmed down." Keeping eye contact to a minimum and stepping away to allow your child to calm down can also be beneficial. If your kid is open to it, encourage him to practice self-relaxing methods like steady, deep breathing or other soothing techniques.

Accept your kids' responses and emotions.

It could be helpful for mom and dad to realize that their kid's angry outbursts are not coordinated attempts to disrupt your lives. This requires both external and internal approval of your infant. Recognizing the child's emotions in an instant can aid in preventing the situation from worsening. "We can see you're upset." Perhaps taking a walk outdoors would help you relax." Similarly, as adults, we will be more prepared to cope with these difficult situations if we adopt a positive approach to them. They are an inevitable part of existence, and seeing them as they are would enable one to cope with them more peacefully.

Get help if you have regular outbursts.

Whether your kid has repeated emotional outbursts, it's important to discover the most powerful parenting techniques for dealing with them. We've discovered that as children's ADHD is best managed, their blazing emotional outbursts decrease in severity and frequency.

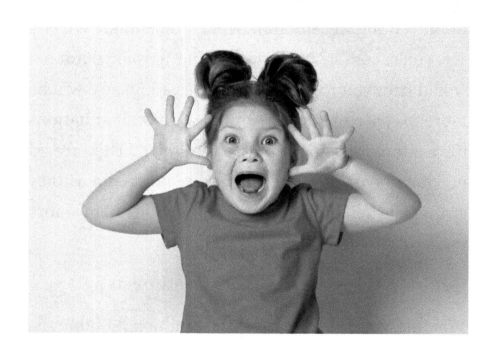

Chapter 4: Parenting with ADHD: Strategies to Help Your Kid

Raising a kid with ADHD isn't like raising a typical child. Depending on the form and nature of your child's symptoms, regular rule-making and household habits can become nearly impossible, so you'll need to take various approaches. It may be difficult to deal with any of your child's ADHD-related habits, but there are opportunities to make life simpler. Parents must accept that kids with ADHD have brains that are functionally different from other children's brains. While kids with ADHD still can learn what is and is not acceptable, they are more susceptible to impulsive behavior as a result of their disorder. Fostering the growth of a person with ADHD requires you to change your behavior and learn to manage your child's behavior.

The first phase in your child's care could be medication. Behavioral strategies for treating a child's

ADHD effects must still be in effect. You will help your child conquer self-doubt and limit negative behavior by adopting these instructions. You're not lonely if you find raising a teen with ADHD to be overwhelming at times. Getting any additional training might help a lot. According to research, meditation and emotional intelligence preparation will strengthen the parent-child partnership as well as your teen's developmental outcomes. Researchers looked at the parenting techniques that resulted in better results for ADHD children and teenagers. Good parenting habits, such as guidelines, rituals, caregiving, and positive stimulation, were linked to healthy child activities. When adults used extreme physical punishments and shouting, ADHD signs and habits became usually greater. Adolescents profit from a multimodal recovery intervention developed by a team that involves the teen, their parents, teachers, and health professionals, much as they did as children. It may be difficult to live with a kid or adolescent who has ADHD or ADD.

However, as a father, you will assist your child in overcoming everyday obstacles, channeling their energies through constructive activities, and bringing greater calm to your home. And the more you resolve your child's issues and the more regularly you do so, the more likely they are to succeed in adulthood. Executive skill deficiencies are common in children with ADHD, including the capacity to consider and prepare ahead, concentrate, manage emotions, and complete activities. That means you'll have to step up as the executive to provide additional support while your child develops executive skills on his or her own. While the effects of ADHD may be exasperating, it's vital to note that your child is not behaving maliciously whether he or she ignores, annoys, or embarrasses you.

4.1 Help your child with ADHD - Stay focused and organized

Follow a routine.

To support the kids with ADHD, recognize and fulfill goals, it's important to assign a period and a location for each. Meals, homework, games, and bedtime routines can all be easy and routine. Before going to sleep, have your child spread out his or her clothing for the next morning, and make sure that anything he or she wants to carry to school is in a designated place, ready to catch.

Use clocks and timers.

Consider putting clocks all over the place, including a large one in your child's office. Allow ample flexibility for your child to complete his or her responsibilities, such as assignments or getting dressed in the morning. Use a timer to keep track of homework or transitional periods, such as when you're wrapping up a game and going to sleep.

Simplify your child's schedule.

While it is beneficial to limit idle time, a child with ADHD can become more overwhelmed and "wound up" if there are numerous after-school events. Based on the actual child's ability and the needs of specific tasks, you will need to make changes to the child's after-school obligations.

Create a quiet place.

Be sure your kid has their own quiet, private room. A patio or a nursery would do, as long since it's not the same location where the infant takes a time-out.

Do your best to be neat and organized.

Set up your house in a neat and orderly manner. Ascertain that your child understands that everything has its proper location. If far as practical, led by the example of neatness and order.

Avoid problems by keeping kids with ADHD busy.

Idle time for children with ADHD can aggravate their signs and cause chaos in the home. It's critical to keep a kid occupied without overburdening him or her.

Enroll your child in an activity, an art class, or a musical instrument lesson. Easy games to use the child's time can be organized at home. Helping you prepare, playing a strategy game with a sibling, or painting an illustration are examples of these activities. Try not to waste so much time watching TV or playing computer/video games. Unfortunately, television and computer games are becoming more offensive, which could exacerbate your child's ADHD symptoms.

Encourage movement and sleep.

Children with ADHD have a lot of resources to expand. Competitive sports and other active activities will help them channel their energies in a positive way while still allowing them to concentrate on basic movements and skills. Physical exercise has many advantages, including improved attention, reduced stress and anxiety, and increased brain development. The fact that exercising contributes to healthier sleep, which in turn will reduce the effects of ADHD, is more significant for children with concentration deficits. Choose a sport that your kid would love, and that is a good fit for their abilities. Softball, for example, is not the ideal sport for children with concentration issues because it involves a lot of "free time." Individual or squad sports that need regular movements, such as basketball and hockey, are safer choices. Children with ADHD can profit from martial arts or yoga training, which improves mental control while still exercising the body.

4.2 Benefits of "Green Time" and Sleep for Kids with ADHD

Spending quality time in nature is beneficial to children with ADHD, according to research. When children play in a park of grass and plants, their signs of ADHD are reduced rather than when they play on a paved playground. Take notice of this promising and straightforward approach to ADHD management. Most families have links to parks and other natural environments, even though they live in a city. Participate in this "green period" with your baby, and you'll get a much-needed breath of fresh air.

ADHD and sleep

Sleep deprivation may render someone less focused, but it can be especially harmful to children with ADHD. Kids with ADHD require at least quite enough sleep as their counterparts without the disorder, but they seldom get it. Overstimulation and difficulty falling asleep may result from their concentration issues. The most effective method for combating this dilemma is a constant, early bedtime, but it might not be enough. Test one or more of the following methods to help your child sleep better:

- Limit your child's screen-viewing time throughout the day and encourage him or her to participate in further sports and exercise.

- Take the coffee out of your child's food.

- Make a buffer window for an hour or two until bedtime to reduce activity levels. Find hobbies that are more relaxing, such as drawing, reading, or playing quietly.

- Snuggle with your kid for ten minutes. This will offer a feeling of affection and comfort as well as a chance to relax.

- Fill your child's bed with lavender or other scents. Your child can feel more relaxed as a result of the smell.

- While your child is falling asleep, use calming tapes as background sounds. There are several different options, such as natural noises and relaxing songs. White noise is also soothing to children with ADHD. Place a radio on static or switch on an electric fan to produce white noise.

Set clear expectations and rules

Children with ADHD want guidelines that are clear and easy to obey. Make the family's code of conduct concise and straightforward. Make a list of the laws and post them somewhere so your child can quickly see them. Children with ADHD react especially well to well-organized reward and punishment schemes. It's critical to clarify what would happen if the laws are followed and what will happen if they are violated.

Finally, stick to the system: follow through with a reward or a punishment any time. Bear in mind that kids with ADHD are often chastised when they develop these consistent constructs. Have an eye out for positive behavior and reward it. Since they usually get very little praise, praise is particularly necessary for children with ADHD. Correction, remediation, and concerns about their actions are provided to these youngsters, but there is no constructive reinforcement. Your child's attention, motivation, and impulse regulation will all benefit from a smile, an encouraging comment, or any reward from you. Focus on providing constructive praise for appropriate actions with job achievement, with a few harsh reactions to inappropriate behavior or bad task success as possible. Reward your child for minor accomplishments that you might overlook with a different child.

Help your child eat right.

While food is not a direct trigger of attention deficit, it does and can influence your child's emotional health, which seems to influence behavior. ADHD affects may be reduced by keeping track of what, where, and how much your child consumes. New produce, daily meal times, and avoiding fast food is beneficial to all children. These principles are important for kids with ADHD, whose impulsivity and distractibility can result in missing meals, disordered feeding, and overeating. Kids with ADHD are known for not feeding on a daily basis. Without parental supervision, these children can go hours without eating and then gorge on whatever is available. The physical and mental wellbeing of the infant can be jeopardized as a consequence of this trend. Schedule daily balanced meals or treats for your child no longer than three hours apart to prevent poor eating behaviors. A kid with ADHD requires daily consumption of nutritious food on a physical level, and meal times include a needed break and a predictable routine to the day on a mental level.

- Exclude all junk foods from your house.

- When dining out, avoid unhealthy and sugary snacks.

- Switch off TV programs showing a lot of fast-food commercials.

- Offer your child a vitamin and mineral intake on a regular basis.

Teach your child how to make friends

Simple social experiences are also problematic for children with ADHD. They can have trouble interpreting social signals, speak excessively, interrupt constantly, or become hostile or "overly intense." Their emotional immaturity will set them apart from other kids their age, making them targets for unfriendly bullying. But keep in mind that many children with ADHD are incredibly bright and imaginative, and they can finally find out how to get along with everyone and recognize others who aren't suitable as companions. Furthermore, personality characteristics that irritate parents and teachers can come across as amusing and charming to peers.

4.3 Improving Your Kids' Social Skills

Learning cognitive skills and social codes is difficult for children with ADHD. You will assist your ADHD child in being a stronger listener, learning to interpret people's expressions and body gestures, and interacting in crowds more smoothly.

- Talk to your child about their difficulties and how to make progress in a gentle yet frank manner.

- With your kids, role-play different social scenarios. Exchange positions sometimes and continue to have fun doing it.

- Choose partners for your child that have a common vocabulary and physical abilities.

- At first, just invite one or two mates at a time. When they're playing, keep a careful eye on them and have a zero-tolerance rule for striking, bullying, or shouting.

- Provide time and room for your kids to play, and praise and encourage positive play habits often.

4.4 ADHD and Sports

Is it appropriate for children with attention deficit hyperactivity disorder (ADHD) to participate in sports? And, of course. Consult the child's pediatrician if you're unsure whether or not they're physically fit to participate in a single activity. Although certain aspects of ADHD can cause difficulties, most children with ADHD are willing to participate in sports.

Difficulties children with ADHD experience in sports

Attention regulation

During practices/competitions, these kids can be more easily distracted and lose sight of their sporting duties.

Motivation/persistence

If you have been through a few levels of challenge, the value of sports begins to decline, and all you want to do is have fun. Readiness for exertion causes hyperreactivity and may lead to increased physical inattention deficiency across time with specific deficiencies, further children to become uninvolved and disengaged in the exercise, causing difficulties in school (examples: not wanting to practice individually between organized events; complaining about attending practice.

Emotional regulation

Inattention deficit hyperactivity disorder (ADHD) can also extend to the child's feelings. Consequently, certain children with ADHD are more likely to lash out (which causes some to some) or get distressed when things may not go their way (because of this, some may misinterpret the situation and unable to see the issue they were previously working to fix). Some of these concerns, to a greater or lesser degree, are an expression of the many kinds of issues common to children of certain ages. Even in comparison to other adolescents, though, it has been shown that children with ADHD have these problems persistently.

Why should kids with ADHD play organized sports?

In general, children participate in athletics for the same purpose as all children do. Sports may include physical activity in a controlled environment, often under the supervision of an adult. This is particularly significant because evidence shows that adolescents with ADHD are more likely to be obese, putting them at a greater risk for adult health issues.

Sports can provide opportunities for positive social interactions.

Peers also dismiss children with ADHD because of their attitudes, though evidence suggests that children with ADHD can overstate the consistency of these relationships. Participating in a group, organized activity will help children have more active social interactions and form friendships, particularly if they struggle with unorganized social relationships.

Sports can provide opportunities for children to develop other talents and interests.

Kids with ADHD often struggle in school; athletics may offer chances for achievement in other ways, promoting better self-esteem and, in some cases, keeping teens more engaged in school. Of note, the same may be done about a variety of other non-academic pursuits, such as involvement in the arts and membership in community organizations.

Are some sports better for kids with ADHD?

There is no indication that children with ADHD may be encouraged to participate in such activities simply as they're more inclined to succeed or that the activity would help them in any way. For example, there is no scientific evidence that participating in martial arts is safer for children with ADHD than, perhaps, basketball or soccer. It's worth noting that ADHD is most likely to create difficulties in cases when the kid considers the task boring or unpleasant. As a result, the right activity for a kid with ADHD is probably to be one that they love and are naturally talented at.

94

Are individual or group sports a better fit?

There is no set guideline, and it depends on the child's desires and preferences, as well as the motivation for involving him or her in sports. Individual sports might be preferable for a child who is easily overwhelmed in a community environment or who requires regular input from a mentor to stay engaged, but this may entail foregoing the enjoyable experience of engaging with peers in a team setting. And individual sports (such as being a member of a swimming or tennis team) can provide further chances for meaningful peer experiences.

Chapter 5: ADHD Kids School and Managing Emotions

Each student who has ADHD is special. Some people need assistance in concentrating and avoiding disruptions. Some people need assistance in remaining coordinated. Others need assistance in getting going with their job or completing work that has already begun. Any ADHD students have difficulty remaining seated or functioning quietly. Inquire for your child's ADHD in the school as well as what you say might do to assist your kid with classwork. For children with ADHD, the school may be difficult, so here are few tips to help your kid or teen excel in the classroom. A child with ADHD can face difficulties in the classroom (ADHD or ADD). These students are asked to perform the same things that they find the toughest still, hearing calmly and concentrating—all day long. The fact that each of these children wishes to be able to understand and perform as their unaffected peers are maybe the most frustrating aspect of all. Children with ADD are unable to learn in conventional forms due to neurological deficiencies rather than a lack of desire.

As a mom, you will assist your child in overcoming these deficits and the obstacles that school presents. You should collaborate with your child to develop realistic learning plans for both within and outside the school, as well as talk with teachers on how your kid understands best. The following tactics, when implemented consistently, will help your child appreciate learning, face developmental challenges, and achieve progress at school and even beyond. Since ADHD affects each child's brain differently, each event in the school will be very different. Children with ADHD have a wide variety of symptoms: some tend to bounce off the walls, whilst some daydream endlessly and can't seem to stick to the laws. You will support your child in minimizing some of more of these habits as a mom. It's important to consider how attention deficit disorder impacts various children's behavior in order to choose the best solutions for dealing with the problem. There are a number of simple steps you and your kid's instructor may follow to help your child overcome his or her ADHD symptoms and get on the path to academic achievement. Making school interesting is a great way to hold a child's mind on the task at hand. Using facial motion in a lecture, linking dry information to fun trivia, or making up silly songs to help your child recall specifics will both help your child appreciate learning and also alleviate ADHD symptoms. One thing we want all to understand is that there is no real thing as an "ADHD brain." In other words, in today's hectic environment, almost everybody might benefit from an extra pair of hands when it comes to handling their time, finances, and even relationships. It's just that these tools are more beneficial to people with ADHD. Keeping coordinated is a difficult task, and people with ADHD can need more assistance than most. Don't confuse your ADHD abilities with signs! It's a collection of characteristics and traits that make you more artistic, spontaneous, caring, and enthusiastic than anybody else you meet. Here are a couple of our favorite ADD advantages. ADHD is a medical disease that inhibits a person's capacity to concentrate, pay attention, and control their behavior. This disease is generally diagnosed in infancy by healthcare professionals. Any individuals, though, are not diagnosed until they are adults. ADHD may often result in a person's having a lot of electricity. There is no one-size-fits-all test for diagnosing ADHD. However, depending on symptoms, healthcare professionals may assess children and adults for the disorder. ADHD is a challenging condition to deal with. Since they have difficulty following orders, some people believe those with ADHD are "out of control" or troublesome. Although getting ADHD may cause behavioral issues, it has also been seen to benefit certain people. You should make sure that your child's communication with his or her school is positive and fruitful. Bear in mind that the common goal is to figure out how to better assist your child in succeeding in education. Have an attempt to be relaxed, precise, and above all constructive when interacting with the school, whether by phone, email or in person. A positive outlook will go a far toward when interacting with the school. You must be compliant at home, just as you must be consistent with medication orders. Children with ADHD thrive in predictable settings. This necessitates a sense of order and routine in the household. Will can note that hyperactivity worsens at unstructured hours and that if left unattended, hyperactivity will spiral out of control. You will reduce the chances of hyperactivity intensifying by creating a regimen with some stability. A cohesive system can evolve into healthier behaviors over time. Your child would be able to control their hyperactivity as a result of this. Though you don't need to micromanage, you can maintain a semblance of order.

5.1 Make Learning Fun

Making school interesting is a great way to hold a child's mind on the task at hand. Using facial motion in a lecture, linking dry information to fun trivia, or making up silly songs to help your child recall specifics will both help your child appreciate learning and also alleviate ADHD symptoms.

Helping children with ADHD enjoy math

Children with attention deficit disorder have a tendency to perceive in "concrete" terms. To understand something different, they also want to keep, contact, or participate in an encounter. You will teach your kid that mathematics can be impactful fun—by utilizing games and artifacts to illustrate mathematical principles.

Play games

To render numbers more enjoyable, use memory sticks, dice, or dominoes. Using the fingertips and toes to connect and subtract by tucking them or wiggling them.

Draw pictures

Illustrations, particularly for word problems, may aid in the understanding of mathematical principles by children. Support your child to draw twelve cars from the steering wheel to the trunk if the term issue says so.

Invent silly acronyms

Made up a song or a word that uses the first word of procedure in the right sequence to recall the order of operations.

Helping children with ADHD enjoy reading.

And if reading is a difficult ability for children with ADHD, there are a variety of ways to make it fun. Keep in mind that reading, at the most simplistic stage, entails telling stories and learning fascinating facts, which all kids love.

- Read to the kids. Make reading a relaxing and enjoyable experience for you and your family.

- Make guesses or "bets." Ask the kid what they expect will happen next on a regular basis. "The girl in the tale seems pretty brave—I think she'll strive to rescue her family," says the model.

- Reenact the novel. Allow the child to pick their character and assign one to you as well. Bring it to life with amusing voices and costumes.

How does your kid like to learn?

Learning becomes a lot more enjoyable for children as it is presented in a manner that makes it easier for them to absorb. If you know how your kid with ADHD understands better, you will design engaging lessons that are also educational.

- Talking and listening are the most effective ways for auditory learners to read. Have these kids sing a favorite song when reciting facts? Allow them to act as though they're on a radio show and collaborate with others on a regular basis.

- Reading or observation are the perfect ways for visual learners to understand. Allow them to experiment with various fonts on the screen and research with colored flashcards. Allow them to scribble or sketch their thoughts on a piece of paper.

- Physical contact or action as part of a tutorial is well for tactile learners. Provide jellybeans as counters and costumes for playing out pieces of literature or culture for these pupils. Enable them to create collages with clay.

Tips for mastering homework

Homework can be dreaded by all children, but for a father/mother of a kid with ADHD, it is a gold mine. Academic work completed outside of the curriculum allows you, as a parent, to directly help your kids. It's a moment where you should help your child at school in the place where you both are more at ease: your own living space. With your help, kids with ADHD will use homework time to practice not only mathematical problems or writing reports but also the organizing and study skills they'll need in the classroom.

Helping a child with ADHD get organized

Whenever it comes to organization, a new start may be beneficial. And if the school year hasn't started yet, take your child shopping for school items like files, a multi-ringed binder, and color-schemed dividers.

Assist the kid in filing his or her papers into the new structure.

- Create a homework folder with completed homework and color-code files to arrange loose documents. Teach your kid how to register properly.

- On a regular basis, assist your child with organizing their possessions, including backpacks, folders, and even wallets.

- Keep an additional collection of homework and other supplies at home if necessary.

- Teach your child how to create and utilize checklists, ticking off tasks when they complete them.

Helping a child with ADHD get homework done on time

Understanding principles and being more prepared are two positive moves, but homework must still be done in one evening and submitted on schedule. With interventions that offer a stable framework, you can help a kid with ADHD get to the finish line.

- Set out a schedule and place for work that is free of distractions such as clutter, cats, and television.

- Enable the child to take a ten-to-twenty-minute break every fifteen to twenty minutes.

- Teach a solid awareness of time by using an analog clock and timer to track homework completion.

- Set up an assignment routine at school: designate a location where students can conveniently locate their completed homework and choose a regular period to send in work to the instructor.

Encourage exercise and sleep.

Physical exercise boosts brain development and enhances attention. It also contributes to more sleep and may help to alleviate ADHD effects in children with ADHD.

Help your child eat right.

Daily healthy meals and snacks, as well as a reduction of junk and sugary drinks, may better control ADHD symptoms.

Take care of yourself, so you're better able to care for your child

Don't forget about yourself. Eat well, exercise regularly, have enough sleep, cope with stress, and seek out face-to-face help from friends and family.

5.2 ADHD Management Tools

One thing we want all to understand is that there is no real thing as an "ADHD brain." In other words, in today's hectic environment, almost everybody might benefit from an extra pair of hands when it comes to handling their time, finances, and even relationships. It's just that these tools are more beneficial to people with ADHD. Keeping coordinated is a difficult task, and people with ADHD can need more assistance than most.

Task planner and calendar

Aside from the apparent benefit of recalling appointments and deadlines, using this method on a regular basis aids you in accomplishing two goals:

- Visualize time passing, make it "real" — this is a difficult challenge for many individuals with ADHD.

- Overcome "major project overload" by breaking down larger projects into smaller ones and arranging them over time.

Writing stuff down will also make you feel more ambitious, and it helps you to physically cross things off your list to see how much you've progressed.

Key chain pill container

Taking medicine on time may be difficult for anybody, but it can be almost unbearable for those with ADHD. Although you should set a reminder to keep your pills in the same spot to provide some consistency, you never know when life could throw you a curveball. Always provide a supply of drugs on hand in case of an emergency. Cielo pill holder is slim, unobtrusive, and very convenient. As a result, the pills will follow you everywhere you go.

Command center

Set aside a room, ideally close to the entrance, for a:

- A whiteboard should be used to convey essential information.

- Create a family calendar

- Keys, papers, handbags, kids' backpacks, library books, incoming dry cleaners, and other essentials may be dropped off and picked up here.

Charging station

Here's an important component to consider when it comes to command centers. Why waste 30 minutes every morning making yourself and everybody else in the house insane searching for your laptop or phone, only to be found with a dead battery?

he Pomodoro Technique

The word "pomodoro" means "tomato" in Italian, but you don't need around red timer to use this method. Any timer would suffice. Setting a time limit is one way to coax yourself out of procrastination and onto a mission.

Jar of Successes

It's simple to become frustrated, particularly in the early stages of diagnosis and care. Two steps forward, one backward step may sound like progress. A loss will depress your outlook and self-esteem if you don't have an aggressive solution in place, and that can lead to a mindset of "why try?" Make a list of accomplishments, big or tiny, including "A classmate praised me for recognizing her" or "I finished a paper in record time!" After that, put them in a pan. This is your success jar. Dip in and read as required later.

5.3 Strategies to Calm Your Child with ADHD

Highlight the bright aspects of your child's life to make them succeed. Here's how to start forming good habits. Every child is different, and it is these distinctions that make them interesting. As parents, it is our responsibility to instill these distinguishing characteristics in our children and to assist them in achieving any goals they set for themselves. We usually emphasize their positives while trying to downplay their negatives in order to make them succeed. The issues emerge as these extraordinary disparities are seen as deficits. Hyperactivity in a child can seem to be a harmful trait. Although hyperactivity and other manifestations of ADHD will obstruct creativity and attention, they are a part of the child's personality and, if treated properly, can help them develop and flourish. So, what are the strongest methods for calming your ADHD kid and assisting them in achieving success?

Follow instructions

It is your responsibility as a parent to follow up with advice once your kid is diagnosed with ADHD and starts therapy. Consistency is crucial once you believe the medicine for your infant is the right option for all of you. It's crucial to understand because if your child's therapy is performed on an intermittent basis, it's impossible to say if it's working.

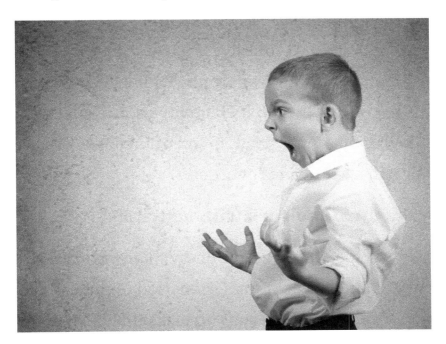

Be consistent with your parenting.

You must be compliant at home, just as you must be consistent with medication orders. Children with ADHD thrive in predictable settings. This necessitates a sense of order and routine in the household. Will can note that hyperactivity worsens at unstructured hours and that if left unattended, hyperactivity will spiral out of control. You will reduce the chances of hyperactivity intensifying by creating a regimen with some stability. A cohesive system can evolve into healthier behaviors over time. Your child would be able to control their hyperactivity as a result of this. Though you don't need to micromanage, you can maintain a semblance of order.

Break up homework with activities

It is disrespectful to ask an individual with ADHD to stay still and be silent for a set period of time. To help them excel, it's best to split up tasks that need a sense of calm into chunks of time. If your child can only do a few minutes of exercise, have them get as much done as they can in that time. They will take a five break after finishing the job to rest, hop about, or do whatever they want before sitting for the next minute or two. This method means that their time lying quietly is effective rather than spent squirming and moving about.

Form the behavior

Shaping is a therapeutic technique that is utilized in cognitive-behavioral and behavioral therapy. Informing, you recognize the action at the current level and use reinforcement to create incremental adjustments. If you decided to add shaping into the prior homework illustration, you might start at six minutes, then break for seven minutes, then break for eight minutes, and so on, until their assignment is finished. You praise your kid as he or she completes the set period of time for daily activity levels. Kind terms, a smile, small sums of money, or an enjoyable outing, later on may all be seen as rewards. This method allows your child to link long cycles of desired energy levels to beneficial outcomes. The periods will extend and grow longer if you are consistent.

Allow them to fidget.

Allow your kids to fidget when performing a job that necessitates a great deal of patience. Allowing them to fidget with a tiny doll, an item of clothing, or a fidget instrument (such as a fidget cube) will increase their concentration and concentration while still reducing their activity rate.

Let your child play before taking on big tasks.

Your child can perform better if they're able to consume off extra energy by playtime until they're asked to sit quietly for an amount of time. For instance, if your kid has been seated throughout the day and bottling up their energy, finishing assignments as soon as they get home might not be the solution. Instead, when they first arrive home, find some mentally challenging, enjoyable things for them to do. Having allowed your kid to participate for half an hour can help them concentrate on their homework more effectively.

Help them practice relaxation.

Learning about coping exercises, using them, and showing them to your child will help them become more conscious of their minds, emotions, attitudes, and hyperactivity. Deep breathing techniques, incremental muscle recovery, mindfulness therapy, imagination, and yoga are examples of these. There are also more relaxing methods available. It will take some trial and error to figure out what the right opportunities are to use these skills, but the outcome will be well worth it.

5.4 Things to Love About ADHD

Don't confuse your ADHD abilities with signs! It's a collection of characteristics and traits that make you more artistic, spontaneous, caring, and enthusiastic than anybody else you meet. Here are a couple of our favorite ADD advantages. ADHD is a medical disease that inhibits a person's capacity to concentrate, pay attention, and control their behavior. This disease is generally diagnosed in infancy by healthcare professionals. Any individuals, though, are not diagnosed until they are adults. ADHD may often result in a person's having a lot of electricity. There is no one-size-fits-all test for diagnosing ADHD. However, depending on symptoms, healthcare professionals may assess children and adults for the disorder. ADHD is a challenging condition to deal with. Since they have difficulty following orders, some people believe those with ADHD are "out of control" or troublesome. Although getting ADHD may cause behavioral issues, it has also been seen to benefit certain people.

The Undeniable Power of ADHD

Be proud of your concentration deficit hyperactivity disorder and all the creativity, wit, drive, and excitement it provides! Read on to learn about some of the strongest characteristics of individuals with ADHD that we all recognize and love.

The Drive of ADD Hyper focus

Hyper concentration, which is a hallmark of ADHD, will be a significant benefit if you can successfully redirect all of your time and focus into work that matters. Many scientists, authors, and artists with ADHD have very fruitful careers, thanks to their capacity to concentrate on a task over long periods of time.

Real ADHD Resilience

ADHD isn't always simple, and we've all had our fair share of setbacks and blunders over the years. People with ADHD, on the other hand, are stronger than ever at getting beyond challenges, adapting different tactics, and going forward. The path at the end of the road is visible. When we slip, we pick ourselves up off of the sidewalk. Through our tears, we smile.

A Sparkling Personality

People with ADHD are brilliant, imaginative, and funny, and they often use self-deprecating humor to show the world that excellence is uninteresting. They've overcome obstacles, discovered new strategies to treat their symptoms, and gained a sense of modesty and self-respect in the process. All of these characteristics combine to create a girl that is a joy to be around and who brightens others' days with her love.

ADD Generosity

Amanda writes that she admires her son's "generosity and determination to please those he cares for the most." He looks out for his younger sister." If it's eating a treat or asking a mate to sob on their back, people with ADHD enjoy making someone smile.

Ingenuity

We may use ADHD imagination in a variety of weird and wonderful ways.

A Strong Sense of Fairness

People with ADHD who have lived with accommodations — or who have struggled without them — realize that "fair" doesn't necessarily imply "equal." They recognize that different individuals need different aspects in order to excel, and they are dedicated to assisting everyone who needs it.

Willingness to Take a Risk

And though it appeared unlikely, Thomas Edison, who had had ADHD, poured his all into inventing the light bulb. It took him over 3,000 attempts to get a working light bulb, but the win was immensely sweet as he had to take a lot of risks; and, even more, failures to get it to work.

Spontaneity

Acting on a whim will also lead to fantastic outcomes. A spur-of-the-moment trip to Great Britain in the middle of a blizzard could lead you to a town you'll fall in love with and eventually relocate to. Learn how to make the most of your spontaneity.

A Great Sense of Humor.

People with ADHD who are well-adjusted have learned to use laughter to deal with stressful circumstances, relieve tension, reinforce relationships, and shift people's minds, among other things.

Constant Surprises

Finding the money (or clothing or a delectable snack) that you had forgotten about adds to life's fun surprises. Who knows what you're going to find next?

Last of the Romantics

"Add pzazz to romantic interludes" with "spontaneity, outside-the-box imagination, and heightened energy," all characteristics of people with ADHD. Adults with ADHD are notorious for lavishing attention on their friends and never losing faith in the force of passion, particularly though their marriages reach a snag.

Engaging Conversational Skills

One thing is certain: there is never a dull moment when you have ADHD! Your continuously spinning mind is constantly directing you towards new topics of discourse and important questions; uncomfortable pauses in the discussion are almost non-existent.

Compassion

Those with ADHD are recognized for their sympathy toward others and ability to lend a hand, despite the fact that we frequently suffer in college or in social settings without proper support. Anyone would rather have a kind, collaborative kid than a smartass who achieves straight as without trying.

Superstar Creativity

Among the popular individuals with ADHD are chef Alexis Hernandez, Justin Timberlake, and comedian Howie Mandel, to name a few. People with ADHD are always articulate and imaginative, as these well-known figures demonstrate, and the disorder can only hold you back if you allow it.

A Different Perspective

Everyone appears to be an "ADHD specialist" these days, and the media often presents the condition in a negative light. You should still be around to correct negative views and spread information whether you live with the disease — or whether you parent a kid that does. Your personal knowledge and unique outlook on the circumstance might be enough to persuade others to change their mind!

Contagious Motivation

It is infectious to get a lot of steam. Those around you would be motivated to achieve their objectives if they see your ambition, enthusiasm, and talent for thinking beyond the box.

Personality strengths of people with ADHD

While not all with ADHD have the same behavioral characteristics, there are certain personal qualities that may render getting the disorder a benefit rather than a disadvantage. These characteristics include:

Being energetic

Some people with ADHD appear to have an infinite supply of resources that they can turn into progress on the sports field, in school, or at work.

Being spontaneous

Some ADHD patients may turn their impulsivity into spontaneity. They might be the life of the group, or they might be more receptive to doing new ideas and breaking away from the standard.

Being creative and inventive

Living with ADHD will have a unique outlook on life and inspire people to treat activities and circumstances with care. As a consequence, some people with ADHD can think creatively. Original, imaginative, and innovative are several other terms that may be used to define them.

Being hyper-focused

According to a study, certain people with ADHD can become hyper-focused. This causes them to become so engrossed in a mission that they may fail to realize what is going on around them. The advantage is that once an assignment is presented, an individual with ADHD will focus on it before it is completed without losing concentration. An individual with ADHD can need guidance in incorporating these characteristics to their advantage. Teachers, psychologists, psychiatrists, and even parents will help. They will assist those with ADHD in exploring their artistic side or devoting their attention to completing a mission.

Research on the benefits of ADHD

More frequently than not, analysis into the positives of ADHD is focused on anecdotes about individuals who have the disorder rather than actual data. Any individuals with the disease say that it has improved their quality of life. In a small 2006 study, researchers discovered that ADHD sample groups were more creative in executing such activities than their peers who were not diagnosed with ADHD. Researchers challenged participants to draw creatures who existed on a world other than Earth to come up with a modern toy concept. A 2017 research looked at the creative abilities of people with ADHD. Participants in the study were challenged to think of different ways to use a book, towel, belt, and tin can. Those with ADHD and those without ADHD produced about the same number of ideas. The researchers have discovered no variations in imagination between those who took ADHD drugs as well as those who did not. When participants in the research were informed, they could earn a prize, people with ADHD came up with more suggestions than someone without ADHD. Rewards and competitiveness can also be effective motivators for people with ADHD, according to previous studies. These observations lend credence to the notion that people with ADHD are also inventive and imaginative.

Creativity

An individual with ADHD should not have to be at a disadvantage in existence because of their condition. Instead, ADHD may and has helped numerous artists, athletes, and business people succeed. Many individuals with ADHD have hit the top of their respective careers. ADHD is a treatable disorder with a variety of medications designed to help people enhance their attention and behavior. Medication and rehabilitation are examples of both. People with ADHD may improve their attention rate as they are given adaptive approaches to assist with time management and organizing skills.

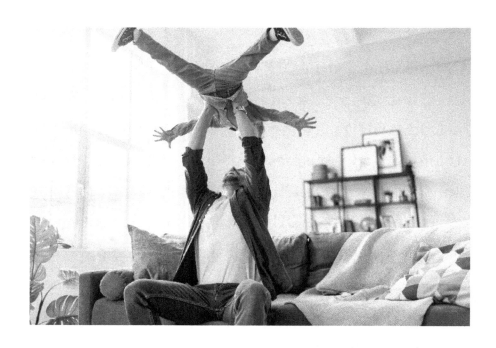

Chapter 6: DBT, CBT, and Somatic Therapy for ADHD

The growing range of non-medical alternatives open to people seeking to change their life is one of the encouraging developments in managing ADHD. Adults who take medicine find that adjunctive treatments, including cognitive-behavioral treatment (CBT) and coaching, will help them properly control the impact of ADHD on their lives. However, while these therapies are successful for certain adults, they are not effective for all. They also demonstrate the paradox of ADHD psychosocial treatment: Behavior modification necessitates advanced skills and tactics, but as we all know, putting them into practice is difficult for people with ADHD. Amanda wanted to find more solutions to her issues. As a result, she turned to dialectical behavior modification, a significant advancement within the CBT family of therapies (DBT). DBT reflects on a person's psychological and mental difficulties. It is not a novel therapy; it first appeared in the early 2000s alongside other CBT-based therapies for adult ADHD.

DBT guides how to develop self-regulation abilities, which could be useful for people who don't adapt to other methods. Before being adapted to handle adult ADHD, DBT was used to treat various psychiatric illnesses. It is the brainchild of The Linehan Institute's president, a professor of psychology at the University of Washington. DBT was created to help people with borderline personality disorder cope with social upheavals, like self-harming habits, including cutting (BPD). Unpredictable mood changes and reckless habits, chaotic interactions, acute stress responses, and a persistent likelihood of self-harm and suicide are also symptoms of BPD. If your kid has been diagnosed with ADHD, your doctor has either spoken about or administered ADHD drugs.

You may have now discovered that behavioral counseling, also known as behavior change, may be beneficial. Keep in mind that these two treatments are not mutually exclusive choices when you strive to find out the right therapy for your boy. In reality, when it comes to resolving ADHD behavior issues, they always function well together. Medication treatment itself, as well as medication and behavioral therapy together, culminated in the largest change in children's ADHD symptoms, according to the National Institute of Mental Health. Furthermore, the hybrid therapy was the most effective in reducing ADHD-related oppositional tendencies as well as other aspects of coping, such as relationships with parents and educators. If you want behavioral treatment instead of medicine because you choose a non-medical solution, your child is too early for medication, or medication has negative side effects, your child will develop emotional, academic, and behavioral skills that can help him manage ADHD over his life. Most children aren't diagnosed with ADHD until they're in kindergarten, but if you think your kid has it until then, it's almost always beneficial (and never harmful) to handle him behaviorally as if he has it. Most people nowadays understand that their minds and bodies are connected in some way.

The area of somatic psychotherapy is concerned with the feedback process that exists between the mind and the body, as well as the aspects in which one continually reminds the other. Physical experiences are as essential to somatic therapists as perceptions and emotions are to talk therapists. Initially, the holistic fusion of body consciousness with classical psychotherapy was utilized to address PTSD by dwelling on the feelings of the body rather than reliving a stressful experience. This method has now been broadened to assist a broader variety of individuals, particularly those with ADHD, in releasing anxiety, apprehension, and rage that may impair their working.

6.1 Somatic Therapy for ADHD

Somatic discomforts can go unaddressed, so ADHD brains don't dwell on uncomfortable problems. Adults with ADHD can benefit from somatic counseling through having to be more aware of body stimuli and can further decrease the level of elevated emotional arousal.

Somatic Therapy Explores the Mind-Body Connection

Most people nowadays understand that their minds and bodies are connected in some way. The area of somatic psychotherapy is concerned with the feedback process that exists between the mind and the body, as well as the aspects in which one continually reminds the other. Physical experiences are as essential to somatic therapists as perceptions and emotions are to talk therapists. Initially, the holistic fusion of body consciousness with classical psychotherapy was utilized to address PTSD by dwelling on the feelings of the body rather than reliving a stressful experience. This method has now been broadened to assist a broader variety of individuals, particularly those with ADHD, in releasing anxiety, apprehension, and rage that may impair their working.

Somatic Therapy for Trauma

A meaningful life requires the desire to feel secure in the company of others. However, the simple comfort may be difficult to come by. Experts in trauma research the fact that trauma creates an indelible mark on both the body and the mind. In self-defense, the hippocampus recalibrates the body's early alert mechanism during a stressful event. Trauma patients are hypervigilant by nature, continuously searching their surroundings for threats. As a result, and though the subconscious removes or distorts distressing thoughts, as it always does, the body recalls the danger in its entirety. As old memories resurface, the body goes into survival mode, causing proper activity to be disrupted. The conscious mind may assume it has the ability to suppress or diminish memories. However, the body keeps track. In helping adolescents with ADHD to regulate their urges, clinicians often utilize somatic approaches to help them become mindful of and restrain the emotional stimuli correlated with impulsivity and violence. However, as individuals mature, therapy normally becomes increasingly intellectualized, with little exposure to bodily stimuli. Research reveals that, relative to people without ADHD, those with ADHD are more prone to develop migraines, stomach problems, body discomfort, and insomnia. Somatic discomforts always go unaddressed, and most ADHD brains may not dwell on uncomfortable problems. Adults with ADHD can begin somatic therapy by learning to be aware of their bodies' sensations. These feelings occur as a stimulus reassures the body it is under threat once again. The body sounds the warning and insists that everything is done.

ADHD and Trauma

According to research, people with ADHD are more likely than most to have undergone abuse at any stage in their life, even though they don't recognize it. It's not quite obvious when a clinical ailment is a reflection of an intrinsic feeling. Many with ADHD often numb themselves from physical discomforts with food, narcotics, sex, unhealthy habits, or workaholism. The somatic treatment gives you both the physical and mental power of the body's anxiety responses.

Somatic Therapy: Key Coping Mechanisms

Here are some of the most effective and simple somatic therapy treatments for reducing the severity of high emotional stimulation:

- Deep belly breathing entails gently inhaling through the nose while causing the chest and belly to expand. Each breath should be held for four seconds before being released through the throat for four seconds. This procedure counteracts the quick, shallow breathing that comes with fear and calms the brain, the brain's emotion control center, by completely extending the lungs.

- Progressive muscle recovery entails sequentially tensing and calming muscle groups as you breathe in and out, starting from your upper body and working your way down to your toes. Strong thinking, such as recalling a happier place, may also speed up the phase.

- Yoga, dancing, exercise, cycling, tai chi, and other forms of activity are excellent for releasing stress retained in the body.

- Meditation requires time, particularly for those with ADHD, but evidence shows that after eight weeks of practice, there is a substantial decrease in stress. It is a method that, like the other interventions, allows for changes in attitude, fear, and concentration.

- Petting a dog or cat has been found to improve dopamine, serotonin, and oxytocin, as well as lower blood pressure, pulse rate, and cortisol, for immediate, short-term relaxation.

Seeing a psychiatrist who uses somatic counseling will help you invest less time treating your depression and more time pursuing a higher standard of life.

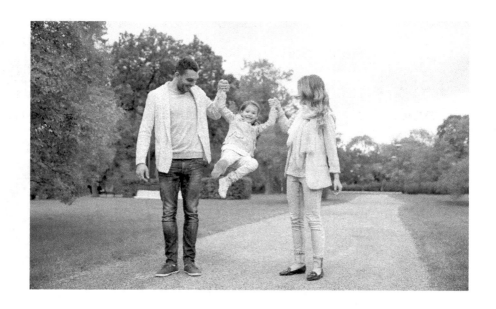

Conclusion

ADHD is a neurological disorder characterized by a history of inattention or hyperactive-impulsive behavior that affects normal life in at least two environments, such as school and home. It affects both boys and girls, as well as individuals from all walks of life. The symptoms mentioned above are representative of the wide variety of signs associated with ADHD, but they vary by subtype. ADHD affects about 8.4% of children and 2.5 percent of adults. When a disturbance in the classroom or difficulties with schoolwork occur, ADHD is often found in school-aged children. Adults may be affected as well. It is more prevalent in boys than in females. It's a behavioral wellbeing condition characterized by a slew of chronic issues, including trouble paying attention, hyperactivity, and impulsive behavior. The mixed form of ADHD affects the majority of infants. Hyperactivity is the most prominent ADHD symptom in preschoolers.

While some unfocused motor movement, inattention, and impulsivity are common, these activities are more extreme and appear more often in people with ADHD. They obstruct or degrade their ability to act professionally, at college, or at work. Some people with ADHD often suffer from another behavioral health issue, such as anxiety or depression. The exact mechanisms of ADHD are yet to be found by scientists. Adult ADHD may cause shaky relationships, weak job or school success, low self-esteem, and a variety of other issues. About the fact that it's called adult ADHD, signs begin in childhood and last until adulthood. ADHD is not often known or identified before an individual is an adult. Adult ADHD signs cannot be as obvious as children's ADHD symptoms. Hyperactivity in adults can decline, but impulsivity, restlessness, and difficulties paying attention can persist. ADHD assessment scales have been used to screen, assess, and monitor the signs of ADHD in both children and adults for almost 50 years.

CPSIA information can be obtained
at www.ICGtesting.com
Printed in the USA
LVHW012319300721
693916LV00003B/243